# THYROID SURGERY HEALING DIET

## Revitalizing Your Recovery And Understanding Dietary Solutions For Hormonal Balance And Muscle Repair

## DR LUCAS KAYCE

# DISCLAIMER

This book about illness and nutrition is not meant to replace expert medical advice, diagnosis, or treatment; rather, it is meant purely for informational reasons. This book's content is founded on broad concepts and recommendations for managing diseases and nutrition.

Before adopting any major dietary or lifestyle changes, readers are recommended to speak with a qualified healthcare provider, such as a licensed physician or registered dietitian, especially if they have pre-existing medical concerns. Everybody has different health demands, so what works for one person might not work for another.

The use of the information provided in this book may have unfavorable repercussions or consequences, for which the author and publisher disclaim all liability. No disease is meant to be identified, treated, cured, or prevented by the information provided.

The book may include contain references to medical literature or research findings; however readers are urged to independently confirm this material and contact reliable sources.

It is important to remember that the fields of nutrition and medicine are always changing, and that new findings could have an impact on the advice offered in this book. As a result, readers are urged to keep up with the most recent advancements in healthcare and, when in doubt, seek professional counsel.

By reading this book, readers agree that they are in charge of their own health decisions and release the author and publisher from any liability arising from the use of the material in the book, whether direct or indirect.

# TABLE OF CONTENTS

# ABOUT THE BOOK

The book "Thyroid Surgery Healing Diet" provides an in-depth explanation of the complex connection between nutrition and the recuperation process following thyroid surgery. This book is an invaluable resource that discusses the critical role that a thoughtful diet plays in supporting overall health, guaranteeing proper thyroid function, and easing the healing process.

The book offers a comprehensive overview of thyroid surgery, including its different kinds, preoperative planning, and postoperative care. These fundamental components lay the groundwork for readers to understand the unique difficulties and possibilities connected to the healing process.

Crucially, the book explores how nutrition affects thyroid function, stressing the complex ways in which dietary decisions affect the course of recovery following surgery.

The book's thorough examination of the Thyroid Surgery Healing Diet Plan is one of its main features.

The concepts, factors to take into account, and doable elements of implementing a diet designed to aid in rehabilitation are covered in this chapter. It gives readers a road map for adjusting their diet according to the kind of surgery they had, stressing the significance of meal timing and frequency in the healing process.

The book will be devoted to elucidating the vital nutrients that are necessary for healing, such as zinc, iron, iodine, and selenium. The author walks readers through a carefully chosen list of thyroid-friendly foods that they can include in their diet, such as whole grains, lean proteins, and fiber. On the other hand, the book offers dietary guidelines that emphasize moderation in the consumption of caffeine and alcohol, advising against goitrogenic meals and processed, sugary foods.

Providing sample meal plans for various stages of recovery and nutrient-rich recipes, the practical aspects of meal planning and dish development are presented in an approachable way. Another chapter emphasizes the significance of supplements and hydration, offering helpful advice on how to stay at optimal levels of hydration and which nutrients are best for recovering from thyroid surgery.

The book discusses the long-term implications of thyroid health beyond the short healing phase. It provides advice on eating a balanced diet, getting frequent checkups, and modifying eating patterns as necessary. With chapters devoted to managing post-surgery difficulties, implementing mindful eating and stress-reduction strategies, and asking friends and family for help, emotional and mental well-being are not disregarded.

The "Thyroid Surgery Healing Diet" is a priceless tool for people traveling the challenging road to recovery following thyroid surgery. The book gives readers the information and resources they need to maximize their recovery and promote long-term thyroid health by fusing medical insights with useful nutritional advice.

# CHAPTER ONE

THYROID SURGERY HEALING DIET OVERVIEW

## CONCERNING THYROID SURGERY

The thyroid gland is a butterfly-shaped organ in the front of the neck that can be removed entirely or in part during a medical procedure known as thyroid surgery. The thyroid is an essential organ that regulates several body processes, such as energy production, metabolism, and hormone balance.

For ailments including goiter, hyperthyroidism, thyroid cancer, or nodules that are uncomfortable or potentially dangerous, thyroid surgery is usually advised.

The patient and the medical staff often give thyroid surgery serious thought before deciding to proceed. An underlying medical issue that is not well treated with medicine or other conservative therapy may need an operation.

Depending on the amount of the gland removed, there are various types of thyroid surgery, including subtotal, total, and thyroid lobectomies.

The healing and recuperation period following thyroid surgery is an important factor. Following thyroid surgery, patients may have transient vocal abnormalities, dysphagia, or stiff neck. A comprehensive strategy is needed to manage these post-surgical side effects, paying particular emphasis to elements that can hasten healing and enhance general well-being.

## DIET IS IMPORTANT FOR HEALING

Notably, nutrition is essential to the healing process following thyroid surgery. The foundation of postoperative care is nutrition, which supports overall health, lowers inflammation and aids in the body's ability to heal. A diet rich in nutrients and well-balanced can help promote tissue healing, strengthen the immune system, and give you the energy you need to recuperate quickly.

Given the significance of diet in the healing process following thyroid surgery, medical practitioners frequently advise patients on dietary recommendations. These recommendations might cover things like getting enough protein in your diet and vitamins and minerals that are necessary for tissue regeneration and wound healing. Sustaining adequate hydration is also essential for general health and helps avoid difficulties throughout the healing process.

Patients are recommended to concentrate on eating a diet low in processed foods and added sugars and high in fruits, vegetables, whole grains, and lean meats. A well-planned postoperative diet can help you acquire nutrients including vitamin A, vitamin C, zinc, and omega-3 fatty acids, which are known to play important roles in the healing process.

Patients and healthcare providers must comprehend the subtleties of thyroid surgery and how it affects postoperative care, especially the role nutrition plays in recovery. Thyroid surgery patients can maximize their healing capacity and improve their general well-being by emphasizing diet as a critical component of their rehabilitation.

# CHAPTER TWO

## COMPREHENDING THYROID SURGERY

## THYROID SURGERY TYPES

The thyroid gland is a butterfly-shaped organ found in the neck. Thyroid surgery, also known as thyroidectomy, involves removing all or part of the thyroid gland. For several thyroid disorders, such as goiter, hyperthyroidism, and thyroid cancer, this surgery is usually advised. Patients undergoing thyroid surgery must be aware of the various types of the procedure, prepare for it, and take care of themselves afterward.

Thyroid surgery comes in a variety of forms, each designed to treat a particular ailment. The three most popular kinds are lobectomy, partial thyroidectomy, and complete thyroidectomy. A total thyroidectomy, which entails the thyroid glands full removal, is frequently advised in cases of hyperthyroidism or thyroid malignancy.

A subtotal thyroidectomy involves the removal of most of the thyroid gland, leaving just a little remnant. A lobectomy, on the other hand, is usually done for benign nodules or tumors that are limited to one lobe of the thyroid gland. It involves removing one lobe of the gland.

## GETTING READY FOR THYROID SURGERY

Healthcare practitioners must perform a thorough evaluation as part of the preparation process for thyroid surgery. Patients may have imaging studies, blood tests, and a comprehensive assessment of their general health before the treatment. Notifying the medical staff of any allergies, prescription drugs, or pre-existing diseases is crucial. Patients may occasionally need to stop taking certain drugs because they may affect the surgical procedure or the healing process. Patients could also be instructed to abstain from food and liquids for a predetermined amount of time before the procedure.

The surgical team and the patient must carefully arrange and coordinate on the day of the procedure.

Preoperative instructions can advise avoiding jewelry or makeup, taking a shower with a particular antimicrobial soap, and dressing comfortably. To keep the patient unconscious and pain-free throughout the surgery, anesthesia is given. Depending on the type of surgery needed, the surgical team skillfully removes the complete thyroid gland or the targeted piece. Patients are observed in a recovery area after surgery to guarantee a seamless withdrawal of anesthetic.

## RECOVERY AND POSTOPERATIVE CARE

Effective postoperative care is essential for a full recovery following thyroid surgery. For a while, patients could feel uncomfortable, swollen, and have trouble swallowing. Medications for pain control are frequently used to treat discomfort. It's crucial to keep an eye on thyroid hormone levels because surgery may have an impact on thyroid function. To preserve a healthy hormonal balance, some patients might need thyroid hormone replacement treatment. Patients are recommended to gradually resume normal activities under the guidance of their healthcare physician, as physical activity may be restricted initially.

 Follow-up appointments are planned regularly to evaluate thyroid function and track the healing process. Particularly for people with thyroid cancer, additional treatments like radioactive iodine therapy may be suggested in some circumstances. The psychological and emotional aspects of recovery are equally significant, and having the assistance of friends, family, and medical experts can enhance the postoperative recovery process.

Comprehending the complexities of thyroid surgery entails being aware of the various kinds of operations, being well-prepared, and providing careful aftercare. A thorough and customized treatment plan is ensured by a collaborative approach between patients and healthcare providers, which ultimately promotes excellent outcomes and optimal rehabilitation.

# CHAPTER THREE

DIET'S IMPACT ON THYROID HEALTH

## THE IMPACT OF DIET ON THYROID FUNCTION

Given that the thyroid gland is primarily responsible for controlling metabolism and other body processes, nutrition has a significant impact on thyroid health. It is crucial to comprehend how nutrition impacts thyroid function to maintain general health. While certain dietary errors may contribute to thyroid dysfunction, a well-balanced and nutrient-rich diet can have a favorable impact on thyroid health.

The consumption of vital nutrients that aid in the synthesis and conversion of thyroid hormones is how diet affects thyroid function. For example, iodine is essential for the production of thyroid hormones. Thyroid conditions including goiter and hypothyroidism can result from inadequate iodine consumption.

Thus, it's essential to consume iodine-rich foods like shellfish, seaweed, and iodized salt to maintain normal thyroid function.

## VITAL NUTRIENTS FOR HEALTHY THYROID

Zinc and selenium are two other minerals that are essential for thyroid support. Zinc contributes to the synthesis of thyroid hormones, while selenium is required for their conversion. Lean meats, sunflower seeds, and Brazil nuts are examples of foods high in these nutrients that can support a healthy thyroid.

## COMMON FOOD MISTAKES THYROID PATIENTS MAKE

However, a few dietary mistakes may have a detrimental effect on thyroid function. Excessive consumption of goitrogens—foods like soy, cruciferous vegetables (including broccoli and cabbage), and some fruits—can disrupt the thyroid's ability to manufacture hormones.

Although most of these foods are nutritious, it's important to eat in moderation, particularly if you have thyroid issues.

Furthermore, thyroid function may be impacted by an imbalance in micronutrients, including iron and vitamin D. Hypothyroidism can result from an iron deficit, and thyroid receptor function depends on vitamin D. Thyroid health can be enhanced by including foods high in iron, such as red meat, and vitamin D, such as fatty fish and fortified dairy products.

Reliance on processed foods with high quantities of refined sugars and harmful fats is a common dietary trap for thyroid patients. These foods may worsen thyroid problems and increase inflammation. Furthermore, consuming too much caffeine might disrupt the body's ability to absorb thyroid hormones, which highlights the need to consume coffee and tea in moderation.

Sustaining thyroid health requires eating a well-balanced diet rich in a range of nutrient-dense foods.

It is recommended that people with thyroid disorders collaborate with medical practitioners or trained dietitians to create customized eating regimens that meet their unique requirements. Thyroid function and general health can be enhanced with routine monitoring and dietary modifications.

# CHAPTER FOUR

THE RECUPERATED THYROID SURGERY DIET

## AN OUTLINE OF THE DIET KNOWN AS "HEALING"

The Thyroid Surgery Healing Diet Plan, which emphasizes nourishing the body and encouraging optimal healing, is essential in helping patients through their recuperation process.

This nutritional approach's main objectives are to minimize discomfort during the postoperative phase, promote tissue repair, and supply vital nutrients.

The Healing Diet is centered on a nutrient-dense, well-balanced diet that emphasizes foods that boost immunity, lower inflammation, and increase energy. Including a range of nutritious foods high in antioxidants, vitamins, and minerals is essential to assisting the body's healing processes. A wide variety of fruits, vegetables, whole grains, lean proteins, and healthy fats are included in this, all of which work together to reduce inflammation and enhance general wellness.

## ADAPTING THE DIET TO THE TYPE OF SURGERY

It is essential to tailor the diet according to the kind of thyroid surgery to satisfy the unique nutritional requirements and probable complications related to each treatment. For example, because the thyroid gland is removed entirely after a total thyroidectomy, patients may need to make long-term dietary modifications.

This could entail following the doctor's recommendations for thyroid hormone replacement medication in addition to keeping an eye on one's iodine intake.

Conversely, individuals who have had a partial thyroidectomy might need to adjust their diet plans depending on the amount of tissue removed and how well the remaining thyroid functions.

# WHEN AND HOW OFTEN YOU EAT

The time and frequency of meals is another important component of the Healing Diet. To ensure a constant flow of nutrients to assist the body's healing processes, a regular eating routine is essential. Frequent eating helps keep blood sugar levels constant, which reduces the risk of energy dumps and encourages a quicker recovery. Eating at the right intervals can also help with drug absorption and digestion, maximizing the body's ability to use nutrients for healing.

When adjusting the schedule and frequency of meals, it is essential to comprehend the tolerance levels and preferences of the individual. Larger, more nutritionally complete meals may be preferred by some individuals, while smaller, more frequent meals may be easier for others to digest. Dietary modifications can be made to the patient's comfort level, guaranteeing that the Healing Diet plan is not only a sensible nutritional plan but also one that is workable and sustainable for the patient's way of life during their recuperation.

By offering a well-rounded and nourishing approach to nutrition, the Thyroid Surgery Healing Diet Plan is intended to assist patients in their recuperation following surgery. The efficacy and efficiency of this nutritional strategy are largely dependent on how it is customized based on the type of surgery and how often and when meals are eaten. Patients can improve their overall well-being and speed up their healing process during the crucial post-thyroid surgery recovery time by adopting these notions.

# CHAPTER FIVE

CRUCIAL ELEMENTS FOR REMEDY

## THYROXINE AND ITS HEALTH

Because it is a vital component of thyroid hormones, iodine plays a critical function in preserving normal thyroid health. Iodine is necessary for the thyroid gland to produce hormones like triiodothyronine (T3) and thyroxine (T4), which are essential for controlling metabolism and maintaining general body functioning. Iodine shortage can cause thyroid dysfunction, which can result in goiter or hypothyroidism. Iodine-rich foods like seafood, seaweed, and dairy products must be a part of the diet to guarantee that the body gets enough of this important vitamin for healthy thyroid function.

## SELENIUM: AN ESSENTIAL ITEM

Another necessary mineral for thyroid function is selenium, which is involved in the transformation of T4 into the more active hormone T3. To help with this conversion process, selenium functions as a cofactor for enzymes, which helps to regulate thyroid function overall. A balanced hormonal profile and the prevention of thyroid problems depend on consuming an adequate amount of selenium. Whole grains, seafood, poultry, and Brazil nuts are good sources of selenium. Maintaining a balanced selenium consumption is crucial because too much of it might have negative consequences.

## IRON, ZINC, AND OTHER ESSENTIAL NUTRIENTS

Zinc and iron are among the essential elements that are essential to the healing process, along with iodine and selenium. Zinc has a role in several physiological processes, such as DNA synthesis, wound healing, and immunological response. Additionally, it aids in the preservation of epidermal integrity and supports the appropriate operation of enzymes. Zinc can be obtained from diet, mostly from meat, legumes, nuts, and seeds. Conversely, iron is necessary for the synthesis of hemoglobin, the protein that carries oxygen throughout the blood. Fatigue and a weakened immune system can result from anemia, which is caused by low iron levels. Foods high in iron include fish, chicken, red meat, and fortified grains.

Sustaining the body's general healing processes requires eating a well-balanced diet rich in these vital nutrients. The interactions among iodine, zinc, selenium, and iron highlight the complex network of dietary needs that support good health. To support the thyroid and other physiological systems to promote healing and prevent shortages, it is essential to ensure that an appropriate intake of these nutrients is obtained through a varied and nutrient-rich diet.

# CHAPTER SIX

ITEMS TO ADD TO YOUR DIET

## FOODS GOOD FOR THE THYROID

Keeping the thyroid healthy is essential for general health because this little gland, shaped like a butterfly, is essential for controlling metabolism. You can promote ideal thyroid function by eating a diet rich in foods that are beneficial to the thyroid. Seaweed, iodized salt, and seafood are examples of iodine-rich foods that are vital because iodine is needed for the synthesis of thyroid hormones.

Moreover, selenium, which is present in turkey, sunflower seeds, and Brazil nuts, aids in the transformation of thyroid hormones into their active form.

Zinc, vitamin B12, vitamin D, and other vitamins and minerals are also essential for thyroid function. Lean meats, dairy products with added nutrients, and fatty fish are good sources of these nutrients.

Furthermore, antioxidants in fruits and vegetables—especially spinach, tomatoes, and berries—can improve thyroid function by reducing oxidative stress and inflammation.

## INCLUDING FIBER AND WHOLE GRAINS

To maintain a healthy weight, stabilize blood sugar levels, and support digestive health, whole grains, and dietary fiber are essential. Selecting whole grains rather than processed grains guarantees a greater consumption of vital nutrients and fiber. Rich in fiber, foods like quinoa, brown rice, oats, and whole wheat promote satiety and facilitate digestion.

Additionally, fiber lowers blood sugar by delaying the absorption of glucose. Those who are trying to control their weight or have diabetes may find this to be especially helpful.

Eating a diverse range of fruits, vegetables, legumes, and nuts will guarantee that your diet is full of both soluble and insoluble fiber, which will help your digestive system function as a whole.

## TRIM PROTEINS TO PROMOTE MUSCLE REPAIR

When it comes to muscle repair and fitness, eating a diet high in lean proteins is essential. As the building blocks of muscles, proteins are essential for the reconstruction of tissues following physical exertion. Lean protein choices, such as fish, turkey, tofu, lentils, and chicken breast, supply you with the essential amino acids without adding too much-saturated fat, which is a drawback of some high-fat protein options.

For those who exercise regularly, getting enough protein in their diet is crucial because it promotes muscle growth and repair.

A well-rounded intake of essential amino acids is ensured by including a variety of protein sources in your diet, which supports total muscle recovery and helps you maintain a healthy body composition.

The promotion of optimal health necessitates a well-balanced diet rich in whole grains, lean proteins, and foods that are friendly to the thyroid. Making dietary decisions that take these components into account promotes general health and physical fitness as well as thyroid function, intestinal health, and blood sugar regulation.

# CHAPTER SEVEN

ITEMS TO STEER CLEAR OF

## FOODS THAT CAUSE GOITER AND THEIR EFFECTS

Goitrogens, which are found in some foods, can affect thyroid function and the body's capacity to absorb iodine, which is essential for the synthesis of thyroid hormones. Brussels sprouts, broccoli, cabbage, cauliflower, kale, and other cruciferous plants are among the fruits, vegetables, and plants that contain goitrogens.

Despite the many health advantages of these foods, people who have thyroid conditions, such as hypothyroidism, may need to use caution when consuming them. Cooking can frequently lessen the goitrogenic effects because heat degrades these substances. However, those who have thyroid issues have to think about speaking with a medical expert to find out how much is right for their particular situation.

# REDUCING SUGARY AND PROCESSED FOODS

Processed and sugar-filled foods are often associated with a wide range of health problems, from diabetes to cardiovascular disease and obesity. These foods frequently have high concentrations of artificial additives, harmful fats, and refined sugars.

Eating processed meals can cause blood sugar levels to surge and plummet quickly, which can cause mood changes and energy swings. Furthermore, consuming too many processed and sugary meals is linked to a higher chance of getting chronic illnesses. Better general health can be achieved by eating a diet high in whole, unprocessed foods including fruits, vegetables, lean meats, and whole grains.

Reducing the amount of processed and sugary foods consumed can help people control their weight better, have more energy, and be at a lower risk of developing several health problems.

# MODERATION IN ALCOHOL AND CAFFEINE

Commonly consumed substances that can affect one's physical and mental health when consumed in excess are caffeine and alcohol. Caffeine, which may be found in coffee, tea, and some energy drinks, has been linked to some health advantages when consumed in moderation, but too much of it can have detrimental effects as well, like insomnia, elevated heart rate, and increased anxiety. Comparably, moderate alcohol use may improve the heart in certain ways. However, excessive alcohol use is associated with several health problems, such as liver disease, heart difficulties, and a higher risk of accidents. Both alcohol and caffeine should be consumed in moderation, keeping in mind each person's tolerance level and underlying medical issues. Getting professional advice can offer tailored suggestions on the best ways to consume these drugs, particularly for people with underlying health issues.

# CHAPTER EIGHT

## RECIPES AND MEAL PLANNING

## EXAMPLE MEAL SCHEDULES FOR VARIOUS REHAB STAGES

Planning meals is essential for helping people get through different stages of recovery, whether they are recovering from a disease, surgery, or any other health-related difficulties. Meal plans that are customized for varying stages of rehabilitation guarantee that dietary requirements are satisfied, fostering mending and general well-being. It's crucial to concentrate on nutrient-dense, readily digested foods throughout the early stages. At this point, soups, broths, and easily digested proteins like lean meats or plant-based substitutes might be included in a meal plan. Including a range of vibrant veggies in your diet gives you vital vitamins and minerals that support healing.

Making the switch to a more varied and balanced diet becomes crucial as recovery advances. This could entail adding more fruits and vegetables, whole grains, and lean proteins. For this intermediate stage, quinoa, roasted vegetable medley, and grilled chicken or tofu could be the meal plan of choice. Consuming foods high in antioxidants, such as leafy greens and berries, can help the body mend itself even more.

It is also important to encourage adequate water during all stages of recuperation.

The meal plan can be further varied to incorporate a wider variety of nutrients in the last stages of recuperation. Whole foods high in omega-3 fatty acids, such as nuts, seeds, and fatty fish, can help lower inflammation and promote general health.

For this stage, grilled salmon, a side of quinoa, and a colorful salad with a variety of veggies can be the meal plan of choice. A well-rounded and nourishing diet is ensured during the latter phases of recovery by incorporating a variety of protein sources, complex carbs, and healthy fats.

# RECIPES PACKED WITH NUTRIENTS FOR HEALING

Recipes high in nutrients are crucial for promoting recovery and giving the body the building blocks it needs to mend itself quickly. A soup made with vegetables and chicken bones is one such recipe. This soup is easy to digest and aids in boosting gut health because it is full of vitamins, minerals, and collagen from the bones. Furthermore, a combination of vital nutrients may be found in recipes that include lean meats like grilled chicken or tofu and a variety of vibrant veggies.

A smoothie bowl made with mixed fruits, leafy greens, and Greek yogurt can be a tasty and healing option for a nutrient-dense breakfast. This dish helps with general recuperation by offering a combination of antioxidants, fiber, and protein. A quinoa salad with different veggies, chickpeas, and a lemon-tahini dressing is an additional choice.

Rich in fiber, healthy fats, and plant-based proteins, this dish promotes healing and increases energy levels.

Consuming meals high in anti-inflammatory components is essential for healing. Cooking using items like ginger, turmeric, and fatty fish can help lower inflammation. For instance, a baked salmon meal marinated in turmeric and ginger has anti-inflammatory properties in addition to omega-3 fatty acids.

## ADVICE FOR MEAL PLANNING AND BATCH COOKING

Meal planning and batch cooking are great tools for keeping a steady, wholesome diet, particularly while recovering from an illness. Selecting dishes that are simple to portion out and scale up for later meals is a crucial piece of advice. Batch cooking is a great way to prepare foods like stews, casseroles, and soups since they freeze well and develop flavor over time.

Appropriate storage is essential to batch cooking success. Meals will stay fresh and tasty if you invest in high-quality airtight containers or freezer-safe bags. It is simple to keep track of what is available and when it was made when containers are labeled with the date and contents.

Efficient meal preparation requires planning. Set aside some time every week to plan your meals, compile a shopping list, and prepare your items ahead of time. Assembling meals during the week can be greatly shortened by washing, cutting, and portioning grains, meats, and veggies. To add variation without increasing the number of components to prep, think about utilizing adaptable items that may be used in many recipes.

Cooking can also be streamlined by using kitchen appliances like sheet pans, Instant Pots, and slow cookers. These gadgets are excellent for cooking big quantities of food and enable hands-off cooking. In the long run, batch cooking and meal planning can be more sustainable if you try several cooking methods and establish a schedule that suits your tastes and timetable.

# CHAPTER NINE

## DRINKING WATER AND TAKING SUPPLEMENTS

## HYDRATION'S CRITICAL ROLE IN THE HEALING PROCESS

Hydration affects several physiological processes that aid in healing, making it an essential component of the healing process. Maintaining blood volume and circulation, which guarantees that nutrients and oxygen are delivered to cells and tissues efficiently, depends on enough fluid intake. Maintaining adequate hydration during the healing phase aids in the body's general detoxification process by supporting the elimination of waste materials and pollutants. Furthermore, proper immune system function is promoted by a well-hydrated body, which strengthens the body's defenses against infection.

Hydration becomes even more important during the recovery phase following surgery, such as thyroid surgery. Surgery might result in increased fluid loss, so it's critical to stay hydrated to avoid complications and encourage a quicker recovery. Dehydration can make wounds take longer to heal and can make recovery after surgery more painful. Therefore, to promote the body's natural healing mechanisms, those having thyroid surgery should emphasize drinking plenty of water regularly.

## SUGGESTED SUPPLEMENTS FOR RECUPERATION AFTER THYROID SURGERY

A topic of consideration is the significance of supplements in the recovery process following thyroid surgery, addition to water. Some supplements can speed up the healing process and lessen any surgical side effects.

Given the effect of thyroid surgery on thyroid function, special supplements are frequently advised for the recovery period following thyroid surgery. These could include omega-3 fatty acids, which are well-known for their anti-inflammatory qualities and can aid the body during the healing process, and vitamin D, which is important for the immune system and bone health.

Calcium is another essential nutrient for healing from thyroid surgery. The parathyroid glands may occasionally be impacted by thyroid surgery, which can cause abnormalities in the regulation of calcium. As a result, taking calcium supplements could be essential to preserve good bone health and avoid problems brought on by a calcium deficit.

## SPEAKING WITH A DIETITIAN OR NUTRITIONIST

Individual needs may differ, so it's vital to remember that speaking with a medical expert—especially a nutritionist or dietitian—is strongly advised. These experts may evaluate each patient's distinct requirements for supplements by taking into account their dietary choices, specific health issues, and any post-surgery demands. To maximize the healing process and reduce the risk of problems, a nutritionist or dietitian can offer individualized advice on the right kinds, amounts, and timing of supplements.

Seeking advice from a nutritionist or dietitian is especially advantageous for patients after thyroid surgery because they can handle nutritional concerns in addition to supplementation and hydration. These experts are capable of creating a thorough nutrition program that enhances general health, facilitates recovery, and supports long-term well-being. A nutritionist or dietitian can provide insightful advice and useful tactics to improve healing and maximize the postoperative journey by taking into account each patient's unique food preferences, constraints, and surgery-related difficulties.

# CHAPTER TEN

CONTROLLING HORMONES AND WEIGHT

## HORMONE BALANCING WITH DIET

Effective weight management is greatly influenced by the connection between hormone balance and nutrition. Hormone levels can be affected by specific diets, which can therefore affect energy storage, metabolism, and overall body composition. For example, eating a diet high in fiber, whole grains, and lean proteins can help control insulin levels, which will help to maintain stable blood sugar levels and prevent the body from gaining too much fat. Flaxseeds and fatty fish are good sources of omega-3 fatty acids, which support the synthesis of anti-inflammatory hormones and help maintain hormonal balance.

Furthermore, adding phytoestrogens from foods like flaxseeds and soy products can aid in balancing the body's estrogen levels. These substances derived from plants function similarly to estrogen and may lessen the signs and symptoms of hormonal abnormalities. Additionally, since vitamin D is involved in the synthesis of several hormones, it is essential for hormonal health to maintain sufficient levels of nutrients through diet and sun exposure.

## KEEPING YOUR WEIGHT FROM CHANGING AFTER SURGERY

Following surgery, weight swings can be a typical problem that requires a systematic approach to manage post-surgical weight. Maintaining a nutrient-dense, well-balanced diet that aids in the body's healing process is crucial. Lean proteins, like those found in fish, chicken, and lentils, can help maintain muscle mass during the healing process. Sufficient protein consumption is necessary for tissue repair.

Additionally, since overeating can result in unneeded weight gain, it is imperative to focus on portion management and mindful eating. A range of vibrant fruits and vegetables should be included because they not only supply vital vitamins and minerals but also help you feel fuller without consuming too many calories. Equally vital is hydration, which promotes healing and helps regulate hunger.

Furthermore, it is advised to resume slow and increasing physical exercise after surgery. Walking and mild stretches are examples of low-impact activities that can improve circulation, stop muscular atrophy, and help with weight management. Before starting any post-surgery fitness program, it is imperative to speak with medical professionals to make sure it is appropriate for your unique healing needs.

## EXERCISE SUGGESTIONS FOR CONVALESCENCE

Exercise is essential to the healing process since it promotes better general health and helps with weight management. People should initially concentrate on low-impact activities to prevent overstretching their recovering tissues. Mild exercises like swimming, walking, or stationary cycling can improve circulation, lessen inflammation, and encourage a phased return to exercise.

Strength training becomes increasingly important as the healing process advances. Resistance training promotes long-term weight control, speeds up metabolism, and aids in the rebuilding of muscle mass. Exercise regimens should be tailored to the specific surgery and degree of fitness of each individual, under the direction of medical professionals or rehabilitation specialists.

Additionally, putting a focus on flexibility exercises helps improve joint mobility and avoid stiffness. Stretching exercises and yoga can be very helpful when you're recovering. Regular exercise and healthy eating habits support a comprehensive strategy for maintaining weight and enhancing general health while recovering.

# CHAPTER ELEVEN



## HANDLING EMOTIONAL DIFFICULTIES FOLLOWING SURGERY

Having surgery may be a very demanding experience, both mentally and physically. In addition to recuperating from the actual surgical treatment, managing a variety of possible emotions is another common aspect of the recovery process.

Identifying and resolving these emotional obstacles is essential for fostering general well-being. During their recuperation, patients may feel afraid, vulnerable, or frustrated.

The efficient management of emotional issues can be facilitated by coping skills such as mindfulness, relaxation techniques, and open communication with healthcare experts.

# TECHNIQUES FOR STRESS REDUCTION AND MINDFUL EATING

There is a well-established link between eating habits and mental health. A more aware and balanced approach to food consumption is promoted by mindful eating, a technique that is based on mindfulness and encourages people to pay attention to the sensory experiences connected to eating.

By encouraging a better relationship with food, incorporating mindful eating into one's routine might help reduce stress. In addition, methods of reducing stress including progressive muscle relaxation, deep breathing, and meditation can be very helpful in controlling the psychological effects of stress.

By developing a greater awareness of their emotions and learning how to handle everyday stressors more skillfully, these techniques help people improve their emotional and mental health.

# ASKING FRIENDS AND FAMILY FOR SUPPORT

Having social support is essential for preserving emotional and mental health, particularly in trying situations. Seeking out friends and family for assistance during difficult times may be consoling, empathetic, and motivating. Opening up to loved ones about one's feelings and ideas creates a supportive environment that can aid in emotional healing. A person's general well-being can be enhanced by the practical help, sympathetic listening, and simple company that friends and family can bring. Stronger support systems are fostered when people in these connections can openly communicate their needs and feelings, which is made possible by effective communication.

Promoting emotional and mental well-being involves a variety of interrelated activities, such as practicing mindful eating and stress-reduction techniques, asking friends and family for help, and managing emotional difficulties following surgery. These techniques highlight how crucial it is to treat mental and physical aspects of health to get a whole sense of well-being. Through the integration of these strategies into their everyday lives, people can improve their ability to withstand stress, develop a positive outlook that promotes their general mental and emotional well-being, and increase their resilience.

# CHAPTER TWELVE

## EXTENDED THYROID HEALTH

## SUSTAINING A NUTRITIONAL PLAN AFTER REHABILITATION

Long-term thyroid health depends on eating a balanced diet. The thyroid gland is essential for controlling several body processes, such as hormone balance, energy production, and metabolism. For the thyroid to work at its best, a well-balanced diet full of vitamins, minerals, zinc, and iodine is essential. Consuming foods high in these nutrients, such as dairy products, nuts, seeds, and seafood, helps support the thyroid glands general health.

Adopting dietary practices that support continued thyroid health is crucial, even after recovering from certain thyroid problems. In addition to supporting thyroid health, a diet high in fruits, vegetables, lean meats, and whole grains also helps ensure that the body is receiving a balanced diet. Antioxidant-rich foods, such as leafy greens and berries, can help fight oxidative stress and inflammation, which can have a detrimental effect on thyroid function.

## FREQUENT INSPECTIONS AND SURVEILLANCE

Long-term thyroid health requires routine monitoring and examinations. Regular thyroid function tests allow medical experts to evaluate the thyroid's function and identify any problems early on. These tests measure thyroid hormone levels (T3 and T4) as well as thyroid-stimulating hormone (TSH). Long-term thyroid health is ensured by monitoring thyroid function, which enables prompt intervention and treatment plan modifications.

## MODIFYING DIET AS NECESSARY

Maintaining long-term thyroid health dynamically involves making necessary dietary adjustments. Depending on their unique requirements, people with thyroid disorders, such as hypothyroidism or hyperthyroidism, may need to adjust their diets.

For example, people with hyperthyroidism may need to restrict their iodine consumption, whereas those with hypothyroidism may benefit from iodine-rich diets. Working together with a medical professional or a qualified dietitian can assist in customizing the diet to meet each person's needs and treat any dietary excesses or deficiencies that may affect thyroid function.

In addition, dietary modifications could be required in reaction to changes in lifestyle, such as pregnancy or age. For instance, the thyroid is subjected to greater demands during pregnancy; hence dietary intake needs to be carefully considered. Thyroid function may be impacted by aging, and dietary adjustments may be necessary to support the thyroid glands evolving requirements.

Preserving thyroid health over the long run necessitates a comprehensive strategy that goes beyond curing particular ailments. Ensuring the thyroid gland functions at its best throughout life requires a diet that is nutrient-rich, well-balanced, and flexible enough to change depending on demands and life stages. Regular checkups are also essential. People can actively contribute to the longevity and vitality of their thyroid health by giving these factors priority.

www.ingramcontent.com/pod-product-compliance
Lightning Source LLC
Chambersburg PA
CBHW060808260726
48660CB00002B/839